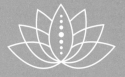

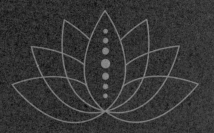

365 DAYS OF

yoga

DAILY GUIDANCE FOR A
HEALTHIER, HAPPIER YOU

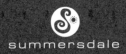

summersdale

365 DAYS OF YOGA

Illustrations – p.8 © VectorPlotnikoff/Shutterstock.com; p.42 © researcher97/Shutterstock.com; all other illustrations © Anna Khramova/Shutterstock.com

An Hachette UK Company
www.hachette.co.uk

Summersdale Publishers Ltd
Part of Octopus Publishing Group Limited
Carmelite House
50 Victoria Embankment
LONDON
EC4Y 0DZ
UK

www.summersdale.com

Printed and bound in the Czech Republic

ISBN: 978-1-78783-641-9

Substantial discounts on bulk quantities of Summersdale books are available to corporations, professional associations and other organizations. For details contact general enquiries: telephone: +44 (0) 1243 771107 or email: enquiries@summersdale.com.

To ....

From ....

introduction

At the centre of yoga is you. Yoga helps you to build harmony between your body, mind and spirit to create a calmer, stronger, healthier and happier you.

If you are a beginner, pace yourself and take things slowly. Yoga is not a competition. It does not matter who can get themselves tied into the tightest knot, or who can hold a position the longest; it is about finding your equilibrium and pace. Nothing is rushed, movement is slow, breathing is long and deep and relaxation is integral to your practice.

Observe your body at all times and respond to how you feel. Strength and stamina build over time, so move away from discomfort or pain in your muscles. Repeat a stretch as many times as

you feel is right for you and always do the same stretch on both sides of your body to keep it balanced. Keep comfortable; remember: yoga is a joyful practice.

Yoga is best practised on a non-slip yoga mat and with bare feet. If you have any concerns with regards to your health, or if you are pregnant, always seek advice from a medical professional or qualified yoga teacher.

This book is a springboard into the year ahead, full of daily inspirations, healthy living tips, suggested yoga poses and stretches to help you take each day at a time. This is a gift for you.

january

Before and after your practice, relax in Corpse to still the body. Lie on your back, feet relaxed and apart, arms away from your body, palms facing up. Focus on your breath to still your mind.

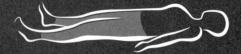

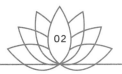

02

The most important pieces of equipment you need for doing yoga are your body and your mind.

RODNEY YEE

03

Whenever you find yourself standing still, practise Mountain. Inhale: engage your legs and thighs, stabilize your core, lift through your chest. Exhale: roll your shoulders back and pull them down the spine.

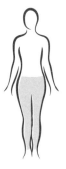

Yoga breathing involves inhalation and exhalation through your nose. The tiny hairs in your nasal passage naturally filter the air before it enters your lungs. Bring this awareness into everyday breathing as you inhale clean air into your body.

The symbol *om* (the word is pronounced "a-au-m") represents what is understood to be the vibrational sound of the universe.

In yoga, a posture or position is called an *asana*. Synchronized with your breathing, every *asana* should be entered, held and exited with control. Practise your favourite *asana*, slowing breath and movement to gain optimum control.

••• (07) •••

Practise Lotus to calm a busy mind. Sit on the floor and bend your right leg so the top of your foot is resting on your left thigh. Repeat with the left leg, placing it on top of the right. If there's any discomfort, try placing a towel under your knees. Stay in the position for a few breaths.

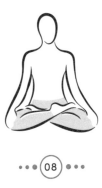

••• (08) •••

Ease tension from your facial muscles at any time in Lion. Inhale: tightly scrunch your face. Exhale through your mouth with a "roar". Drop your jaw, open your eyes wide and extend your tongue.

Start writing a diary dedicated to your yoga practice. This safe place is where you can reflect on your thoughts, feelings and observations in order to develop honest communication with yourself.

Breathe away January blues with a breathing meditation. Inhale for the count of eight, exhale for the count of sixteen. Deeper relaxation is achieved through deeper exhalation.

Sow love, reap peace.
Sow meditation, reap wisdom.

SWAMI SIVANANDA

Release emotional energy stored in your hips by practising Bridge. Lie on your back. Inhale. Exhale: bend your knees and place your feet on the floor. Inhale: push your hips into the air. Hold and breathe for as long as you feel comfortable.

Yoga is the perfect opportunity to be curious about who you are.

JASON CRANDELL

Breathe in Low Lunge to encourage muscle relief in your groin and thighs. Start on all fours. Inhale: bring your left foot between your hands, with toes and fingertips in line. Exhale: sink into your right thigh. If it feels good, you can stretch your arms up above your head. Repeat on the other side.

Your feet carry you everywhere you go. Treat them to a warm foot soak at the end of a long day to show them your loving gratitude.

••• (26) •••

You can use a folded towel to make yourself comfortable during your practice by sitting on it or placing it under your knees. Cover yourself with it during relaxation to retain your body heat.

••• (27) •••

Enjoy a lovely opening of the throat with Fish. Lie on your back and slide your hands, palms down, underneath your buttocks. Press down through your forearms and lift your chest, tilting your head back to bring the crown of your head to the floor. Lower on an exhale.

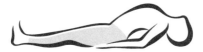

You can't do anything about the length of your life, but you can do something about its width and depth.

ANONYMOUS

•••(29)•••

Observe Three-Part Breathing to empower your everyday breathing pattern. During inhalation feel your stomach rise, then feel your ribcage expand and, finally, feel your chest inflate. As you exhale feel your chest fall, followed by your ribs and then your stomach.

Tune in to your feelings to stay connected with your emotional self. Ask, "How do I feel right here, right now?" Listen to your answer and react appropriately.

Rest your liver; have an alcohol-free week. Monitor any physical or emotional reactions you experience in your diary. You may choose to modify your drinking habits for longer.

••• (18) •••

Follow a sequence of standing body twists to neutralize your spine and to release any pressure. Inhale: raise your hands above your head. Exhale: lower your left hand across the front of your body and your right hand behind you. Feel the twist in your waist and through your torso. Repeat on the opposite side.

**Breathing is one of
the greatest secrets of yoga.
If you practise it with sincerity,
you will obtain healing powers
beyond your imagination.**

BIJA BENNETT

Stimulate your digestion with a Seated Twist. Start in Staff (see page 28) and bend your right leg toward you. Lift it to the outside of your left thigh and bring your left foot close to your right buttock. Exhale as you twist to the right, right hand behind you on the floor and left arm placed on the outside of your right knee, hand to the sky. Hold for a few deep breaths, then repeat on the other side.

••• 21 •••

Use a mantra (*man* meaning mind, *tra* meaning instrument) – a sound vibration that is repeated aloud or in your head – to connect mind with spirit during meditation.

••• 22 •••

Keep your eyes closed throughout your practice to deepen your concentration on your internal world. "See" your body from the inside out.

••• 23 •••

Squeeze your shoulder blades together to energize the area. Inhale: raise your arms above your head. Exhale: lower them behind your back, interlock your fingers and extend your arms. Inhale: bring the heels of your hands together. Exhale: release.

Breathe in Child to ease discomfort in your lower back. Start on all fours. Inhale: stretch your tail bone skyward. Exhale: slowly lower your buttocks to your heels, forehead to the earth. Bring your arms by your side, with your fingers in line with your toes, or stretch them out in front of you.

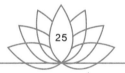

Practice makes the heart grow fonder.

STEPHANIE PAPPAS

Cross-legged, or Happy Seat, is the most popular position for meditation. Place cushions under your knees to make yourself comfortable, allowing your hips to open without strain.

A *mudra* is a hand gesture that seals or locks your energy; it is yoga for your hands.

Bring the tips of the thumb and index finger together on both hands and extend the remaining fingers. This is *Gyan Mudra*, which promotes clarity of mind during meditation.

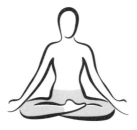

february

Watch something funny or laugh out loud just for the sake of it! When you laugh, endorphins are released, your mood is lightened and your stomach muscles get a gentle workout.

Bring your hands together, leaving a little hollow space between your palms, in peaceful Prayer, *Atmanjali Mudra*, to harmonize left and right brain hemispheres. This *mudra* calms thoughts and creates harmony, peace and balance within oneself.

In any position requiring balance, focus on a fixed point in front of you to enhance your concentration and stabilize your position. This is known as the *drishti* point.

Feel steady and strong in Warrior I. Start in Low Lunge (see page 12). Inhale: straighten and extend your right leg back. Exhale: squeeze your buttocks to stabilize your lower back. Inhale: bring your hands above your head, continuing to breathe here for as long as is comfortable. Repeat, stretching out your left leg.

Treat yourself to a Tibetan singing bowl – a type of bell whose deep, resonant sounds can aid relaxation and reduce stress – and enjoy using it to open and close your daily meditation.

On World Meditation days, which occur on the first Sunday of every month, do a simple sensory meditation. Take a few minutes to notice what you can see, hear, smell, taste and feel. Whenever you slip back into thinking, gently bring your focus back to your senses.

••● 07 ●••

Replace tea and coffee with herbal tea or hot water for a few days this week. See if you notice any difference in how you feel and the quality of your sleep.

••● 08 ●••

Muscle has memory. If your practice has lapsed, do not be deterred. Get back onto your mat, and your muscles will be happy to gently ease back into familiar stretches.

••● 09 ●••

Love your body, learn to accept and be happy with how you look. Move away from judging and celebrate how amazing you and your body truly are.

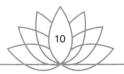

When you listen to yourself, everything comes naturally. It comes from inside... Try to be sensitive. That is yoga.

PETRI RÄISÄNEN

Give your spine and chest a gentle stretch in Sphinx. Lie on your front, forearms flat on the ground with your elbows underneath your shoulders. Lift your upper torso on an inhale, engaging the core to support your spine.

Move in Clock to open your shoulders. Stand with your left shoulder and hip in contact with a wall. Inhale: raise your left arm against the wall to a 12 o'clock position. Exhale: lower it to one o'clock. Continue moving around the clock, breathing alternately in and out on each "hour". Repeat on your right side.

••● (13) ●••

Instead of reaching for the headache tablets, kick off your shoes and rub your big toes, which represent your head in reflexology. Massage them to send healing energy to your headache. Remember to drink plenty of water as headaches can be a result of dehydration.

Gently flex your spine in Cow. Start on all fours. Inhale: tip your tail bone skyward, dip your navel toward the floor, lift your head. Exhale: tilt your head back, look skyward.

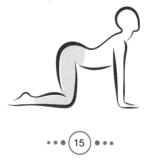

••• (15) •••

Send focused healing energy to an area of discomfort in the body with *Mukula Mudra*. Bring the tips of your fingers and thumb of one hand together, like a bird's beak, and place on the area of unease. Connect and breathe for several minutes.

••• (16) •••

Throughout the day, rotate your ankles one way, then the other to keep your joints warm, flexible and mobile when the weather is cold.

••• (17) •••

Notice how the daylight hours are getting longer in the evening and enjoy the thought that spring is around the corner.

••• (18) •••

Shake, shake, shake to free yourself of an unwanted feeling or negative vibration. Relax your muscles, loosen your joints and shake. Visualize any negative feelings evaporating.

Sit in Staff to lengthen your hamstrings and improve your posture. Sit with both legs extended. Inhale: adjust your position so that your "sit bones" connect to your mat. Exhale: lengthen your spine and place your palms to the earth.

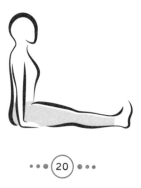

••(20)•••

If you need some support as you build on your flexibility and deepen your practice, invest in a yoga block. You can use it to prop yourself up for floor postures or shorten the distance between you and the ground for standing positions.

••• 21 •••

The quickest way to experiencing the peace inside is to learn to recognize when I am not at peace.

JAMES PATRICK McDONALD

••• 22 •••

Strengthen the soles of your feet to improve standing balances. Inhale: slowly rise onto the balls of your feet. Exhale: lower your heels slowly to the earth. Inhale: rock back onto your heels, lift your toes. Exhale: lower your toes. Repeat at least three times.

Embrace the lightness and joy that yoga ignites. Feel free to smile through your practice and shine!

Find stability in Half Moon. Start in a wide-legged standing position. Lift your arms so they are in line with your shoulders and your chest is broad. Prepare for the posture by turning your right foot out, bending your right leg and transferring your weight onto it. Tilt your body over to the right and start to lower your right arm to the floor. As you do this, allow your left leg to lift, so the movement is like a pendulum. If you can't reach the floor with your hand, use a block. Aim for your left leg to be parallel with the floor, or higher if you can, and stretch your left arm up to the sky. Hold for a few breaths and repeat on the other side.

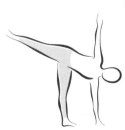

Stroke your face from jaw line to cheeks using your fingertips and light, rapid upward movements. This will stimulate blood flow, creating a warm glow and an instant facelift!

••● 26 ●••

Crying is like laughing; it helps to free and cleanse the soul. Give yourself permission to release your tears and let them flow.

••● 27 ●••

In yoga, breath control is called *pranayama* (*prana* meaning universal energy, *yama* meaning control). Optimizing and controlling your daily breathing patterns will help reduce stress levels and maintain a healthy body and mind.

Strengthen your arms and shoulders in Plank. Lie on your front, hands palms down with your wrists below your shoulders. Tuck your toes and lift your body off the mat, using either your forearms or your palms for support. Hold the position for a few breaths, thinking about pulling the heels of your feet together. Build your stamina by holding the pose a little longer each day.

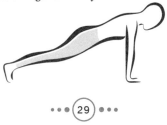

••• 29 •••

This day only appears once every four years. View it as an opportunity to do something special for yourself in your practice and make the most of the additional day - perhaps by doing yoga outside to enjoy the fresh air and seeing if you can spot the first signs of spring.

march

Notice a detail in nature: the spiral of a snail's shell, the pattern in the veins of a leaf or the delicacy of a petal. Remind yourself you are part of nature.

Yoga is not a competition. Don't compare yourself to others, or to the flexible people you see modelling the poses online or in books. Your practice is personal, and by embracing yoga you have already won!

Table Top is a simple pose which is great for bringing a sense of balance and strength to the whole body at the start of a yoga session. Come onto your hands and knees. Your hands should be directly under your shoulders and your knees underneath your hips. Keep your shoulders back and lengthen the spine.

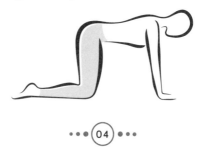

•••(04)•••

Spring is in the air! Open windows and doors to remove stale energy. Allow the fresh spring breeze to flow through your house and refresh your space.

If you have been sitting for a long time and your muscles have been inactive, take a mindful moment to prepare your body for action. Before you move, think, "I am ready," and inhale as you stand. Fill your lungs with new energy to prepare yourself to move.

Place an object (for example, a stone or pen) on the end of your finger to explore your sense of balance. Challenge yourself to move around without the object falling off your finger.

···• 07 •···

Choose today to try a meat-free diet for the next three days, week or however long suits you. Get your protein through eggs, nuts, tofu, cheese or beans. Note any differences in how you feel in your yoga diary.

••• •••

Declutter your space to make more room in your life, both physically and mentally. Target an overloaded wardrobe, the packed-to-within-an-inch-of-its-life garden shed or an overflowing kitchen drawer.

••• •••

You cannot control the results, only your actions.

ALLAN LOKOS

••• (10) •••

Remind yourself during the day to roll your shoulders back and pull your shoulder blades down your spine to encourage good posture. Keep your chest lifted to promote a feeling of confidence.

Relax your lower back in a gentle Reclined Twist. Lie on your back. Inhale. Exhale: bend one or both knees to your chest. Inhale. Exhale: lower your knee(s) to the left, turn your head to the right. Repeat on the other side.

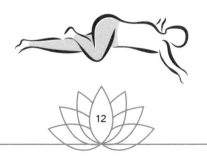

Yoga does not ask you to be more than you are. But it does ask you to be all that you are.

BRYAN KEST

Listen to your body. If you are recovering from an injury, refrain from participating in a full practice to allow sufficient time for your body to heal. Focus instead on stretches or gentle exercises that don't put any weight or pressure on the affected area.

Ignite personal energy in Energy Ball. From a cross-legged position, inhale to prepare yourself. Exhale: bring your knees to your chest and wrap your arms tightly around them. Lower your nose to your knees. Keep still and as small as you can while you continue to breathe.

••• 15 •••

Listen carefully to how you speak to yourself to nurture a positive mindset. Change your expression from "I can't" to "I can" and reap the rewards.

●●● (16) ●●●

Lie still in this gentle hip-opening meditation to bring relaxation to the ligaments around your hips. Lie on your back and join the soles of your feet together, knees out wide. Breathe and relax into the position. Hold for as long as you feel comfortable.

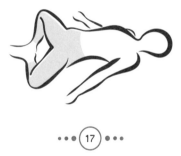

●●● (17) ●●●

Draw imaginary circles with your hip, knee and ankle joints to keep them flexible and loose. Balance on one foot, freeing the opposite leg to explore small and large circular movements in each joint.

••• (18) •••

At the beginning of your practice today, set yourself an intention. Are you going to focus on smooth and even breathing? Maybe you want the session to clear your mind and bring you peace. Or perhaps you'd like to move through the poses with gratitude for what your body can do. See how different intentions change your experience.

19

**Be a lamp to yourself.
Be your own confidence.
Hold to the truth within
yourself as to the only truth.**

BUDDHA

Massage your lower back in Happy Baby. Lie on your back. Inhale: bring your knees to your chest, direct the soles of your feet skyward. Grab your feet with your hands, allowing your knees to relax and fall out to the sides. Exhale: gently rock side to side.

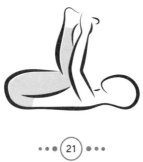

••● 21 ●••

Spring-clean your yoga mat by spritzing it with a mixture of water and a few drops of tea tree essence oil, which has natural disinfectant qualities.

Practise Frog to help open up your hips. Start in Table Top position (see page 34). Slowly move your knees away from each other, to the side, and breathe deeply. As your body lowers, move from your wrists onto your forearms and try to keep your feet as close together as possible. Hold the position for a few breaths. If you start to feel any discomfort, release your body from the pose.

•••（28）•••

Notice the difference in evening light as the clocks go forward by an hour for summertime!

•••（29）•••

Set yourself a new goal to challenge your mind and body, such as working toward achieving a new *asana*.

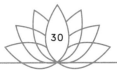

30

In the midst of movement and chaos, keep stillness inside of you.

DEEPAK CHOPRA

••●(31)●••

If you've been hunched over a desk all day, try this opening stretch. Lie face-down on the ground and bend your arms so they make right angles, palms down. Keeping your right hand on the floor, roll onto your right side so your right ear comes to the ground. Lift your left leg and place your left foot flat on the floor behind you. You'll feel a deep stretch in the front of your right shoulder. Repeat on the other side.

april

•••◉ **01** ◉•••

Try a simple breathing technique to help still and quieten the mind. Inhale for the count of six, exhale for the count of twelve. Come back to your breath if your mind wanders.

•••◉ **02** ◉•••

Explore the meaning of yoga — unity. Start in Happy Seat (see page 19) and bring the soles of your feet together. Wrap your hands around them and focus on the point of union between left and right.

••• 03 •••

Yoga is a light, which once lit will never dim. The better your practice, the brighter your flame.

B. K. S. IYENGAR

••• 04 •••

Be your best friend, not your enemy. Smile in the mirror and tell yourself, "I love you."

••• 05 •••

After each *asana*, or a longer flow of practice, breathe deeply until your heartbeat is stabilized to allow your blood circulation to become steady.

Before you go to sleep, reflect on your day. Look for the positive in all your experiences and give thanks.

Give a powerful stretch to the whole body in Downward Dog. Start in Plank. Inhale. As you exhale, lift your tail bone skyward, push back with your hands and stretch your heels toward the earth. If the pose is too hard on your wrists, come down onto your forearms.

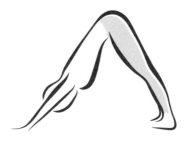

**Remember the emphasis
on the heart. The mind lives
in doubt and the heart lives in
trust. When you trust, suddenly
you become centred.**

OSHO

••• 09 •••

Switch off your TV, give yourself a break from
social media and spend a night in with a yoga book
from the library. Research your favourite *asana*.

••• 10 •••

Swing your arms to shift blocked energy. Stand in
Mountain (see page 7). Inhale and exhale as you
swing your arms forward and backward. Clap your
hands whenever they come together.

Look out for rainbows in the sky during April showers to remind you of the wonders of nature. Let the colourful light fill you with happiness.

To trim your waist and strengthen your core, inhale and lift your hands above your head. As you exhale, lower your left arm by your side and gently lean to the left. Repeat on the opposite side.

●●● 13 ●●●

Remove stale air to make way for oxygen-rich air with *Kapalbhati* breathing. Inhale a long, silent breath through your nose and allow your stomach to swell. Exhale: contract your stomach muscles and release the breath through your nose sharply. Repeat several times, breathing in and out through your nose. Do this for no more than 10 to 20 seconds at a time to begin with, and stop if you ever become dizzy.

••• (14) •••

Change the way you look at things, and the things you look at change.

WAYNE DYER

••• (15) •••

Invigorate your energy flow in Seated Forward Bend. Begin in Staff (see page 28). Inhale: raise your hands above your head. Exhale: unhinge from the hips and fold forward, keeping your spine straight. Hold your shins, ankles or toes depending on your flexibility and breathe for as long as you feel comfortable.

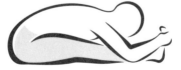

••• (16) •••

Create some time for yourself. Book a day off work and indulge in a "free to be me" day by doing whatever you feel like doing.

••• (17) •••

Turn your hands so that they are palm up with fingertips pointing toward each other. Then place one hand on top of the other, and touch your thumbs together in *Dhyana Mudra*. This hand gesture means meditation, and provides completeness during still moments.

••• (18) •••

Be present in every moment today. Remember: you have a choice in everything you do.

To revive tired legs, lie on your back with your buttocks against a wall and your legs vertically up the wall. Place a rolled-up towel under your lower back for extra support. Inhale: stretch your legs upward. Exhale: rest your arms out to the sides, palms up. Breathe deeply and hold for as long as you feel comfortable.

Write a letter or send a card through the post to say hello to someone who is dear to you.

Try Revolved Side-Angle for an instant energy boost. Start in Warrior I (see page 21) with your right leg forward, then bring your palms to Prayer (see page 20), resting them on your chest. Inhale and lengthen your spine, crown to the sky. Exhale as you twist to the right, resting the outside of your left elbow on the outside of your right knee. Hold for several deep breaths, then release on an exhale and repeat on the other side.

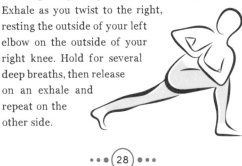

Today, do your practice in controlled, super slow motion to draw your attention to how your body feels.

Observe spring bulbs, such as tulips and daffodils, as they shoot up from the dark. Think about the abundance of energy and natural information that lets each bulb know it's springtime!

Hold and breathe in a Squat to open up your groin and release compression to the lower back. Start in Mountain (see page 7). Inhale: adjust your feet so they are slightly wider than your hips and move your weight onto your toes. Exhale: bend your knees and slowly lower buttocks to heels.

may

01

Connect with your inner spirit in Warrior II. Start in Mountain (see page 7). Inhale: step back with your left foot and turn it out slightly. Exhale: bend your right knee. Inhale. Exhale: extend your right arm forward, your left arm behind you, so they're straight out and parallel to the ground. Hold for as long as you feel strong. Repeat on the other side.

02

We can learn a lot from each other: share your knowledge.

Breathe to centre yourself in
Thunderbolt. Kneel with your
buttocks resting on the soles of your
feet. If it's more comfortable for you,
place a towel under your thighs. Rest
your palms on your knees and
lengthen through your spine.
This is a comfortable seated
position for meditation.

The muscles in your body are interconnected. They
twist, turn, contract, lengthen, tense and relax.
Visualize your muscles softening and loosening
during relaxation to let go of tension.

Let food be thy medicine and medicine be thy food.

HIPPOCRATES

If your stomach feels uncomfortable, incorporate some extra twists into your practice to detox and boost your digestive system.

Nurture a plant. Water it regularly, keep it in sunlight and watch it grow daily... just like you.

13

Remember, it doesn't matter how deep into a posture you go – what does matter is who you are when you get there.

MAX STROM

14

Fold into Standing Forward Bend to allow blood flow to revitalize your brain. Start in Mountain (see page 7). Inhale. Exhale as you fold forward from your hips, aiming to connect your palms with the earth. Bend your knees slightly if your legs feel tight.

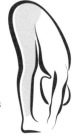

For a day or two after your practice, regardless of your fitness level, you may feel gentle aches in your muscles where they have been working hard. Feel encouraged. These sensations will pass and they actually show that your muscles are getting stronger!

Rub your scalp with small circular movements, as if you are washing your hair, to stimulate nerve endings under your scalp and to help soothe tension.

●●● 17 ●●●

Eat slowly to aid digestion. Put your knife and fork down and take breaks between mouthfuls, allowing time for your taste buds to savour the array of flavours in your food.

···●(27)●···

Treat your body to a massage. Comment in your diary on the feelings you experienced and the sensations you noticed before and after your massage.

···●(28)●···

Make a light snoring sound at the back of your throat as the air enters your body, in *Ujjayi*, or Ocean Breath. Tap into *Ujjayi* breathing to empower your inhalation and tone your epiglottis, which lies at the base of your tongue.

···●(29)●···

Indulge and have fun; book a yoga retreat, or make your own – turn off all screens for the weekend and commit to three yoga sessions a day: at sunrise, before lunch and as the sun sets.

•••(30)•••

When you find peace within yourself, you become the kind of person who can live at peace with others.

PEACE PILGRIM

•••(31)•••

To increase the energy flow in your spine, practise Cat. Start on all fours. Inhale. Exhale: curl your tail bone, arch your back and look toward your navel. Breathe. Hold. Then release. Repeat as many times as you enjoy.

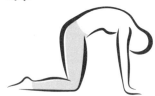

Reflect and observe any changes you have experienced during your yoga journey so far. Perhaps your general energy levels have increased, or maybe you are feeling stronger, calmer, more flexible. Yoga has many benefits; how has it benefitted you?

Be at least as interested in what goes on inside you as what happens outside. If you get the inside right, the outside will fall into place.

ECKHART TOLLE

••• (18) •••

Rub your hands together and gently place your palms over your eyes to create a dark place to soothe tired and irritated eyes. Breathe.

••• (19) •••

Balance in Warrior III to improve circulation. Start in Mountain (see page 7). Inhale: slowly lift your left leg behind you. Exhale: lower your torso so it's parallel to the earth. Stretch your arms forward. Breathe and hold the position for as long as you feel comfortable. Repeat on the other side.

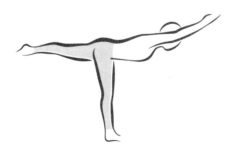

june

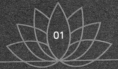

01

When we give cheerfully
and accept gratefully,
everyone is blessed.

MAYA ANGELOU

To build stamina in your abdominal muscles lie on your back and, as you inhale, lift your legs slightly off the floor. Hold and breathe for as long as you feel comfortable. Lower your legs on an exhalation.

••• (03) •••

Life is challenging, full of surprises, and change is inevitable. Yoga can help you embrace life's challenges positively with calmness and flexibility.

••• (04) •••

Cup your hands around your knees and begin to rub round and round, in one direction, then the other. This gentle circular movement warms, relaxes and soothes joints. Give your elbows the same treatment!

••• (05) •••

Visit a lake, fountain, waterfall, river or the sea to experience the relaxing pleasure of all of your senses responding to the nearness of water.

••• (06) •••

Lift into Inclined Plank to invigorate your heart. Start in Staff (see page 28). Put your hands on the ground behind you, fingertips pointing toward your buttocks. Inhale: push your hips into the air. Exhale: extend your toes to the floor.

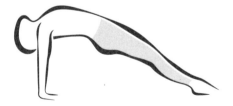

Close your eyes. What can you hear? Meditate on the sounds of summer around you and breathe in the warm air.

•••(08)•••

Balance in Boat to clear your mind. Begin in Energy Ball (see page 38). Inhale. Exhale and, sitting on your tail bone, extend your legs slightly, holding them up in the air straight in front of you. Extend your arms to the front or bring them above your head to deepen the pose.

•••(09)•••

If any good intention has lapsed, recognize this and reset your intentions. Start afresh without guilt or judgement.

Blow on a fully seeded dandelion head and watch the seeds drift away to make a new life elsewhere. Feel comforted that the circle of life is forever working its miracles.

Enjoy a blissful side stretch in Peaceful Warrior. Start in Warrior II (see page 58), left leg forward. Turn your left hand palm up, then stretch back, left arm reaching up to the sky and right hand resting on the back of your right leg. Keep lifting your left arm further to deepen the stretch. Repeat on the other side.

Try the mantra *lam* (pronounced "l-a-au-m") during meditation as an alternative sound to *om*. These sounds are linked to the main chakras to stimulate energy movement. *Lam* is associated with the root chakra and the colour red.

••• (13) •••

In Table Top (see page 34), tuck your toes and lift your knees slightly off the mat, pressing through the palms, for a quick strengthening pose. Hover for a few breaths and then lower on an exhale.

••• (14) •••

Open your arms to the universe and give thanks to Mother Nature.

••• (15) •••

For every minute you are angry you lose 60 seconds of happiness.

ANONYMOUS

••• (16) •••

Supine Pigeon, or Eye of the Needle, offers a satisfying stretch in the hamstrings and hips. Lie on your back, knees bent, and relax your upper body. Cross your right leg over your left thigh, and clasp the back of the left thigh with both hands (your right hand should thread through the gap). Draw the thigh you are holding in toward your chest while pressing your right knee away from you, until you feel the stretch on the back of your right leg. Repeat on the other side.

If you feel uncomfortable at any time during your practice, try slightly softening and bending your knees to avoid overstraining the muscles on the back of your legs or knees. Yoga is about working with what feels good for you, so move away from discomfort and pain when you feel it.

The palms of the hands are powerful sensors of energy. To increase energy flow at any time: inhale, and as you exhale, spread your fingers wide apart and stretch across your palms. Hold for three breaths. Relax your hands on an exhalation.

•••(19)•••

Chop your food finely when you are preparing lunch or dinner to make it easier to chew and to allow nutrients to be more easily absorbed by digestive juices.

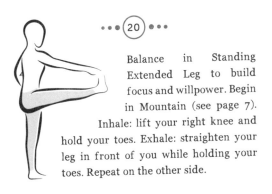

••• (20) •••

Balance in Standing Extended Leg to build focus and willpower. Begin in Mountain (see page 7). Inhale: lift your right knee and hold your toes. Exhale: straighten your leg in front of you while holding your toes. Repeat on the other side.

••• (21) •••

Honour the longest daylight hours of the year with a mindful practice of Sun Salutation at sunrise and sunset. Give thanks to the circle of life. For a basic Sun Salutation, you might want to move smoothly through the following poses: Mountain, Forward Fold, Halfway Lift, Plank, Chaturanga, Upward-Facing Dog or Cobra, Downward Dog, Halfway Lift, Forward Fold, Mountain.

Make a natural scrub to exfoliate your face. Mix a teaspoon of brown granulated sugar with three teaspoons of olive oil. Gently rub the mixture into your skin using small circular movements. Rinse with warm water and pat dry.

••• (23) •••

Connect with the earth. Walk barefoot in the park, bringing your attention to the sensations of the grass under your feet (but watch out for anything sharp).

••• (24) •••

Be open to saying "yes" today. Embrace new opportunities that come your way: actively accept an invitation, an offer of help or an act of kindness.

Combine hula-hooping with yoga breathing to get your energy flowing and your hips moving. Your muscles will be massaged and toned with the circular movement of keeping the hoop in the air, and you will have fun, too!

Sometimes our light goes out, but is blown again into instant flame by an encounter with another human being.

ALBERT SCHWEITZER

Stand in Tree to cultivate focus and balance. Start in Mountain (see page 7). Inhale: place the sole of your right foot on the inside of your left leg (avoiding your knee). Exhale: bring your hands together in Prayer (see page 20), extending upward to reach to the sky if you feel comfortable and balanced. Repeat on the other side. Hold for as long as you feel you are able to.

Before you leap out of bed in the morning, wake your spine gently to avoid straining your lower back. Lying on your back, inhale and bend your knees to your chest. Rotate your ankles in both directions.

When the mind... becomes still by the practice of yoga, then the yogi is able to behold the soul through the purified mind, and he rejoices in the inner joy.

BHAGAVAD GITA

Slowly lower your head to release tension in your neck. Inhale. Exhale and gently lower your head to the left. Inhale and raise your head back to the centre. Exhale and repeat to the right. Inhale and return to centre.

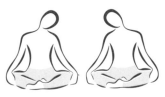

july

Renew energy in your shoulders, especially after heavy physical work, with this standing pose. Inhale: squeeze your shoulder blades together. Feel your muscles compress. Exhale: roll your shoulders forward. Feel the warm rush of blood to this area.

Whenever you practise a posture where your feet are connected to the ground (*Pada bandha*), visualize a triangle of anchor points on the soles of your feet. Focus on your heel, the ball of your big toe and of your little toe. This will create a firm foundation, or rooting, for your feet.

Run cold water over your wrists to cool your body temperature on a hot summer day. Let the water flow over your pulse points and notice the difference in how you feel.

Practising yoga during the day is... about listening inwardly as often as you can for your deepest impulses about what to say, think, or do, or be.

ERICH SCHIFFMANN

••• (05) •••

Practise yoga with a friend; support each other, help each other to make adjustments and give suggestions to help refine your postures.

When you are lying on your back, uncurl and straighten your tail bone to lengthen your spine and feel the extra release it brings.

•••(07)•••

Give yourself an all-over stretch and strengthening exercise with Side Angle. Start in Warrior II (see page 58) with your left foot forward. Rest your left forearm on your left thigh, and extend your right arm over your head, close to your ear. Turn your head up toward the sky. If you want a deeper stretch, extend your left arm down to the floor just inside your foot.

•••(08)•••

Acknowledge a new moon during the month as a manifestation of a new cycle. Allow it to empower the beginning of your own cycle of change.

Apply moisturizing cream to your body to rehydrate your skin after exposure to the sun. Use upward strokes toward your heart to help stimulate the lymphatic circulation.

Strengthen and stretch your legs, hips and pelvis all in one with an Extended Leg Squat. Start in a wide-legged standing position. Bend onto your left leg, turning out the foot as you lower and keeping your right leg straight. Bring your hands to Prayer (see page 20). You should feel a satisfying stretch along your right inner thigh. Hold for a few breaths and repeat on the other side.

Aim to eat a colourful plate of food every day to guarantee a variety of the minerals and antioxidants that are essential for a healthy body.

12

The way to do is to be.

LAO TZU

●●●(13)●●●

Be still in Halfway Lift to strengthen your back while stimulating your internal organs. From a Standing Forward Bend (see page 63), inhale and lift your torso so that it's parallel to the earth, and rest your palms on your shins or thighs. Hold. Release the position as you exhale.

It all comes to this: the simplest way to be happy is to do good.

HELEN KELLER

••• (15) •••

Go green for the day. Drink green-based juices, like spinach or kale. Eat green salad with broccoli to boost your immune system and fill your body with natural goodness.

••• (16) •••

When the moment feels right for you, concentrate on your exhalation in *Charlie's Angels Mudra* to direct spent energy away from your body. Place your index fingers together. Interlock your remaining fingers, cross your thumbs and point your index fingers so stale energy shoots away from your body.

Shelter from the heat of the sun under the shade of a tree to keep cool. Give thanks to the tree for its protection.

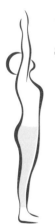

Stretch your waist in Standing Crescent to give additional tone and strength to your stomach muscles. Inhale: bring your palms together above your head. Exhale: bend to the left. Repeat on the other side. Repeat as many times as you like.

Build stamina in your abdominal muscles with Leg Raises. Lie on your back, arms by your sides, palms down. Inhale: lift your leg, directing the sole of your foot toward the sky. Hold for three breaths, lower as you exhale. Raise your legs individually or together.

The attitude of gratitude is the highest yoga.

YOGI BHAJAN

Watch butterflies fluttering about their daily business on a hot summer's day. Bring qualities of their movement – lightness, grace and agility – into your movements during your practice.

••• (22) •••

Release tension in your lower back in a
One-Legged Standing Balance. Stand
in Mountain (see page 7). Inhale: lift
your left knee. Exhale: wrap your
hands around it and bend your elbows to
bring your knee closer to your chest. Repeat
on the other side.

••• (23) •••

Why not place a damp folded cloth over your eyes
when you relax in Corpse (see page 6)? The extra-
dark, cool environment is a perfect way to rest
tired eyes.

••• (24) •••

Remember to remove your watch while you
practise. It is time to breathe and be in the
moment. No need to clock-watch! If you're
worried about losing track of time, you can
always set a gentle alarm.

Try Reverse Table Top to counter any forward bends and open up the front of the body. Start sitting on your mat with your feet on the floor, hands behind you with palms flat on the ground, fingers facing toward you. Inhale and lift your hips, straightening your body as you extend through your arms. Keep your knees at a right angle and pull your shoulder blades together.

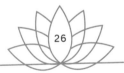

Blessed are the flexible, for they shall not be bent out of shape.

ANONYMOUS

••• 27 •••

Prepare your body for more intense bends and twists with Pyramid. Start in a wide-legged standing position, with your left foot facing the top of your mat and your right foot turned in slightly. Align your upper body and hips to the front leg, shoulders back. Reach both arms behind you and bring your palms together in Prayer (see page 20), fingers pointing up toward your head. Reach your crown to the sky for a few breaths, then on an exhale, fold forward at the hips until your upper back is parallel to the ground. Repeat on the other side.

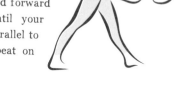

••• 28 •••

Take advantage of a clear night sky bejewelled with twinkling stars. Spend some time stargazing and look out for shooting stars.

To strengthen your buttocks and thighs try Chair. Stand in Mountain (see page 7). Inhale. Exhale, and with knees, ankles and heels together, bend your knees lowering yourself onto an imaginary chair. Bring your hands into Prayer (see page 20).

The blossom of meditation is an expressible peace that permeates the entire being.

SWAMI VISHNUDEVANANDA

Try drinking fresh coconut water to replenish your body, especially after practice. It is a rich source of electrolytes, which are responsible for keeping the body properly hydrated so the muscles and nerves can function properly.

august

Tune in to the gentle noise of summer leaves rustling in the trees. Actively feel the breeze cooling your skin and enjoy the sensation.

Refresh your energy flow by taking regular breaks throughout the day. Inhale: bring your hands above your head and interlock your fingers. Exhale: turn your palms toward the sky. Hold and breathe deeply.

Allow your thoughts to pass through your mind like clouds on a summer day. Breathe into this calm image while you meditate to keep your mind free of distraction.

••• (04) •••

Stand in a Wide-Legged Forward Bend, toes
slightly turned inward, to help unblock a stuffy
head. Inhale: cross your arms above your head.
Exhale: fold forward with your legs straight. Let
your arms and head hang loosely or touch your
fingertips to the mat. Breathe. Remember to work
with how you feel, slightly bending your knees if
you feel any strain.

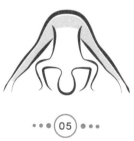

••• (05) •••

Your mind and your body are intrinsically linked.
If muscles are relaxed, your mind is relaxed; if
your mind is tense, your body is stressed. Inhale
for a count of four and exhale for a count of eight
to harmonize both.

Remember: you are your own teacher. Listen carefully to how your body feels and avoid straining. Rather than forcing your body, breathe and relax into a position. Move away from pain and discomfort during any stretch and take things slowly.

Sound the mantra vam (pronounced "v-a-au-m"), associated to the sacral chakra and the colour orange, during your meditation to release energy in the base of your spine to ground yourself and to feel personal connection with your mind, body and spirit.

For a deeper chest stretch in Bridge (see page 11), try clasping your hands together underneath your buttocks and drawing your shoulder blades together.

Most folks are usually about as happy as they make their minds up to be.

ANONYMOUS

Your lungs are like balloons – inflating, deflating, driven by muscular action of the diaphragm. Each lung has approximately 300 million tiny air sacs inside. Visualize each tiny sac filling up and emptying again every time you inhale and exhale to maximize breathing potential.

Go foraging for blackberries in your local area. Use them in a fresh fruit salad or freeze them for winter.

Deepen the stretch in your shoulders as you stand in Wide-Legged Forward Bend (see page 97) by reaching your arms behind your back and holding the opposite arm at the elbow.

If it feels good, you can then lift your elbows up and away from your back to open up the front of the underarms and enjoy a deep stretch.

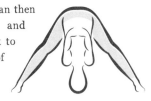

Be creative: invent your own *asana* to personalize your practice.

• • • (14) • • •

Bring the positive virtues of honesty, kindness, compassion, love, understanding and patience into your day to be the best person you can be.

• • • (15) • • •

Celebrate summer. Enjoy eating outside to boost your mood and to absorb energy from the sun. Contact with the sun on your skin produces essential vitamin D, which is good for your heart and immune system.

• • • (16) • • •

To soothe sinuses irritated by a high pollen count, cover your head with a towel and bring your face over a bowl of hot water. Breathe deeply for ten minutes.

The goal is... to experience your own spirituality and the interaction of body and mind in each pose.

ATHANASIOS KARTA SINGH ON YOGA

Practise Locust to strengthen your buttocks, legs, arms and shoulders. Lie on your front. Inhale: extend your arms behind you, hands clasped. Exhale. Inhale: lift your legs and arms. Exhale: lower legs and arms.

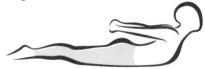

••• (19) •••

Efficient circulation depends on a healthy heart. Practise your favourite *asana* to promote positive energy flow. All *asanas* are beneficial to your mind, body and spirit.

••• (20) •••

Butterfly your knees in Happy Seat (see page 19) to open your hips. Move your knees up and down quickly like a butterfly's wings to encourage energy flow to this area.

••• (21) •••

Avocado is a superfood, packed with healthy fats and high levels of vitamins that are good for your heart. You can also mash the flesh and use it as a face mask. Smear a thin layer directly onto your skin and leave for five to ten minutes to let the goodness be absorbed. Rinse with water and pat dry.

27

Sway your arms from side to side, twisting at your waist and keeping your hips facing forward, to loosen your spine after sitting still on a long journey.

28

I will not be distracted by noise, chatter or setbacks. Patience, commitment, grace and purpose will guide me.

LOUISE HAY

29

If you like to rest or sleep on your side, place a cushion or pillow between your legs to separate your knees – it will help keep your hips aligned and avoid aches and pain.

Develop focus, balance and upper body strength in Crane. Place your hands on the floor shoulder distance apart. Bend your knees and rest them on the backs of your upper arms. Inhale. Exhale and lift your feet. Refrain if your wrists are feeling weak.

Use *Agni Mudra* to improve digestion during your meditation. Connect your thumb and middle finger on each hand, and extend the first, third and fourth fingers away from the palm. Breathe.

september

Re-energize aching shoulders with simple shoulder lifts. Inhale: lift your shoulders toward your ears. Exhale: slide them down. Repeat several times with slow, mindful breaths.

Focus on micro-adjustments available to you during your practice. On your inhalation feel your body expand, swelling with new energy; as you exhale, gently move into the spaces you create in your body.

03

In truth yoga doesn't take time – it gives time.

GANGA WHITE

••• 04 •••

Clean your feet daily, especially before you stand on your yoga mat, to help keep your mat fresh.

••• 05 •••

Prepare your food with your full attention and always let love be a main ingredient. Once your dish is ready to be enjoyed, practise mindful eating and savour each mouthful, chewing slowly and noticing how all your senses are being stimulated.

Organize a fun social gathering to nurture new friendships with fellow yogis in your class.

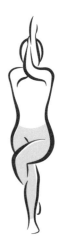

Stand in Eagle to improve your balance. Start in Mountain (see page 7). Inhale: wrap your left leg around your standing right leg. Exhale. Inhale: twist your arms together in front of your body, joining your palms. Exhale: slightly bend your knees and lift your elbows away from your chest. Repeat on the other side.

Whatever you do to one side of your body in yoga, repeat the same movement on the other side to keep left and right balanced.

To think creatively, we must be able to look afresh at what we normally take for granted.

GEORGE KNELLER

···•(10)•···

Brighten up your yoga space. Even if that's just the floor of the living room, you could bring in some objects that make you happy before your practice, such as a crystal or a houseplant. Enjoy the process of planning, preparation and productivity and the added satisfaction of energy well spent.

Have a quiet day to yourself: switch off your phone and avoid the computer and the television. Find solace in your own silence and inner peace.

Sit in Tail Bone Balance to focus your mind. Begin in Staff (see page 28). Bring your knees to your chest. Wrap your arms around them. Inhale and lift your feet off the floor, finding balance on your tail bone. Hold and breathe.

••• 13 •••

Yoga is beneficial to everyone of every size, shape and age. Be gentle with yourself, know your limits and avoid comparing yourself to others.

Concentrate on Backbend in your evening practice to elevate your mood. Keep your chest and heart lifted as you breathe all the way down into the small of your back.

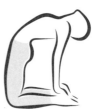

Ultimately spiritual awareness unfolds when you're flexible, when you're spontaneous, when you're detached, when you're easy on yourself and easy on others.

DEEPAK CHOPRA

As autumn settles in, embrace the intensity of colours in the sky at sunset.

Try Thread the Needle to relax your shoulders. Begin in Child (see page 16). Inhale: extend your left arm under and across your body. Exhale. Inhale: raise your right arm skyward, and, as you exhale, slowly lower it to join both hands together.

••• 18 •••

Every day is an opportunity to create change in your life.

Your wrists are made up of eight individual bones, making them delicate parts of your body. To ease the pressure of aching wrists, use your knuckles or fingertips in your practice instead of pressing flat palms onto the floor.

Begin each day as if it were on purpose.

MARY ANNE RADMACHER

••• (21) •••

Pay attention to the abundance of colour in nature as the leaves turn yellow, orange and red, ready to fall. Consider how these changes are part of the cycle of the natural year.

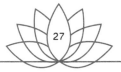

Live each day as if it were your last, without frenzy, without apathy, without pretence.

MARCUS AURELIUS

Deepen your stomach breathing in Corpse (see page 6). Lightly place your hands on your stomach. Inhale and feel your hands rise as your stomach rises. Leave your hands where they are and notice your navel sink toward your spine as you exhale.

••• (29) •••

Be patient with yourself; switch off the critical, negative voice and promote positive thoughts. Negativity eats away at you; positivity serves you.

••• (30) •••

Sitting down, cross your legs one over the other and breathe deeply in Cow Face to increase flexibility in your upper body. Inhale: stretch your hands above your head. Exhale: circle your right hand down and then up behind your back, between your shoulder blades. Bend your left arm over your right shoulder, aiming to join your hands together. Flexibility will come with time and patience.

october

In the West we sit on chairs, causing stiffness and inflexibility in the hips. Bring yourself down to the floor and sit cross-legged instead of sitting on the couch. Notice how upright and relaxed you feel in this position.

In the same way that you make space in your body and mind, try to free up other areas of your life as well. Clean up your phone, for instance, by deleting unnecessary or unwanted messages, contacts and apps.

When you are landing or jumping back from a position, think the words "land lightly", so that you move consciously and mindfully.

To reduce general fatigue in your legs, ankles and feet, lie on your back, with a cushion or rolled towel underneath your knees. Relax with your arms away from your body, palms facing up. Breathe.

Know well what leads you forward and what holds you back, and choose the path that leads to wisdom.

BUDDHA

Eat fresh pineapple to soothe a sore throat. Pineapple contains bromelain, an enzyme that has anti-inflammatory properties as well as many other vitamins and minerals that will help you on the road to recovery.

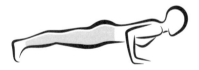

Start in Plank (see page 32) with your heels back and your shoulders directly above your wrists. Keeping your elbows hugged tight into your sides, bend at the elbow to a right angle, bringing your shoulders forward and lowering halfway to the ground. Keep your whole body straight as you work your arms, wrists, shoulders and core.

When did you last replace your bed linen, pillows, toothbrush, towels, underwear or socks? Replace any you have had for a long time; old towels in particular can develop a pungent smell. Try to find a use for the unwanted materials, or donate them to a used clothes bank or charity shop if you can.

Rustle up a delicious spicy vegetable curry for dinner. As well as providing wonderful flavour and aroma, garlic will cleanse the blood, turmeric will flush the liver and cumin has anti-carcinogenic properties.

To help deepen your breathing pattern, visualize the power and strength of ocean waves as they rhythmically roll in and out of the shore.

●●● (11) ●●●

This lovely opening pose provides a deep stretch to your inner thighs and hips. Start in Staff (see page 28), then extend your legs as wide as you comfortably can while keeping the toes pointing up and making sure your hips aren't rolling forward. Exhale as you fold over, engaging your core and taking hold of your big toes or your ankles. Fold deeper into the pose, bringing your forehead toward the mat between your feet, keeping your shoulders back and down.

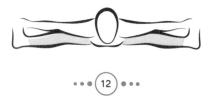

●●● (12) ●●●

Drink ginger tea to boost your immune system and protect your body against colds, coughs and splutters. Add thin slices of fresh ginger to a cup of hot water.

We all wish for world peace, but world peace will never be achieved unless we first establish peace within our own minds.

GESHE KELSANG GYATSO

Practise *Yoni Mudra* to bring concentration and calm to your mind. Close your ears with your thumbs and your eyes with your index fingers. Your middle fingers control your breathing as you alternate closing each nostril and your remaining fingers press your lips together. Observe a sense of tranquillity as you breathe deeply for a few minutes.

••• (15) •••

Set a calming mood to create a soothing environment for your practice. Burn incense or a scented aromatherapy candle, dim the lighting, play gentle meditation music or have a natural object nearby.

••• (16) •••

Enhance your balance, flexibility and energy with Reverse Triangle. Start in a wide-legged standing position, with your front foot pointing to the top of the mat and back foot turned in slightly, both legs straight. Reach your front arm up to the sky, then bend back until your back arm rests on the back of your knee.

Ease stiffness from your neck with a gentle head roll. Inhale to prepare. Exhale: lower your chin to your chest. Inhale: slowly roll your head to the left. Exhale: roll your chin back to your chest. Inhale: roll your head to the right. Exhale: return your chin to your chest.

••●（18）●••

Our emotional and physical needs change constantly; pay attention to how you are feeling, and tap into your emotional self throughout the day for personal harmony.

••●（19）●••

Go for a sauna or Turkish bath to absorb deep heat into your muscles, bones and joints.

One of the most effective hip-opening positions is Pigeon. Start in Downward Dog (see page 48). Bring your left leg forward so your knee comes to the mat just behind your left hand. Lower down so your left heel is opposite your right hip, and your right leg is straight back on the mat. Square your hips. If there is a gap between your left buttock and the floor, place a towel or yoga block in between for support. To deepen the stretch, you can fold forward here and place your forehead on the mat. Repeat on the other side.

Have a complaint-free day! Move through your day without talking negatively. Promote the positive in every situation and focus less on the negative.

••• 22 •••

If you feel exhausted from your day, and only have
a little time for your practice before you are on the
move again, lie on your back and take a moment
in Corpse (see page 6) to regain your equilibrium.

••• 23 •••

No matter how grey it looks, the sky is still blue
above the clouds.

••• 24 •••

Choose the mantra *ram* (pronounced "r-a-au-m")
to stimulate energy flow in your third chakra, the
navel area. Focus on yellow, the colour associated
with this chakra.

••• (25) •••

If you want to conquer the anxiety of life, live in the moment, live in the breath.

AMIT RAY

••• (26) •••

Stretch the entire front of your body in Bow. Lie on your front. Inhale: bend your knees, bringing your feet toward the back of your head. Exhale: reach behind you and hold on to your feet. Inhale: lift your chest and knees. Release as you exhale.

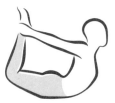

Enjoy a selfless act, known as karma yoga. Donate some of your time and energy today to someone who needs your help, company or support.

28

The tongue is a muscle without which we cannot speak. In a quiet moment roll, curl, extend, twist and push up and down with your tongue to mindfully exercise it.

29

Carve a pumpkin and illuminate it with a candle to create a seasonal atmosphere during your practice. Use the flesh to make a savoury dish, a pumpkin dip or a delicious pumpkin pie.

Calm your mind and reduce stress and anxiety levels by practising Plough. Lie on your back. Inhale: bring your legs above your head. Exhale: lower them slowly to the floor behind you. Hold. Breathe.

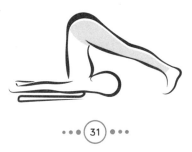

••• 31 •••

As the clocks go back, take notice of the extra daylight in the mornings. Burn a candle to celebrate light.

november

 01

Hang bags of bird-friendly nuts to help hungry birds with their daily quest for food. Winter is a challenging time for them too!

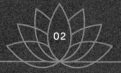 02

Be yourself.
An original is always
worth more than a copy.

SUZY KASSEM

Be strong and stable in Triangle. Stand in a wide-legged standing position. Inhale: swivel your right foot sideways, raise your arms to make a "T" at shoulder height. Exhale: reach to the right, then lower your right hand to the floor. Lift your left arm above your head and turn your head skyward. Repeat on the other side. If you can't reach the floor, use a yoga block to support you.

Use yam (pronounced "y-a-au-m"), the mantra meditation connected to the heart chakra, to open energy flow in the heart. Surround yourself with the colour green, which is associated with the fourth chakra.

••• (05) •••

Stimulate your colon, liver and kidneys while opening your hips in Baby Cradle. Begin in Staff (see page 28). Inhale. Exhale: bend and lift your left knee out to the side, and then cradle your left knee and lower leg in your arms. Gently rock it side to side for as long as you like. Repeat on the other side.

••• (06) •••

Feelings come and go like clouds in a windy sky. Conscious breathing is my anchor.

THÍCH NHẤT HẠNH

••• (07) •••

As soon as you get home, remove your shoes and socks. Move, stretch and flex your toes to liberate them after being restricted all day.

••• (08) •••

Work on overall body strength to improve your general practice. Breathe in Half Plank, resting on your elbows and forearms instead of on your hands. Hold for as long as you feel comfortable.

••• (09) •••

Tension causes muscle fibres to tighten, which can restrict blood flow and lead to the development of sore areas known as "knots". Relax on your back for five minutes or longer with a tennis ball under the knot to help break down the tenderness.

••• (10) •••

Life would be a dull place if we were all the same. Live and let live. Avoid comparing yourself to others, celebrate the differences and be happy to be you.

••• (11) •••

Energize your lower back in Upward-Facing Dog. Lie on your front. Place your hands on the floor below your shoulders. Inhale and push down through the tops of your toes, lifting your chest and lower body off the ground. Roll your shoulders back and down and extend your crown upward to lengthen the spine.

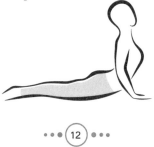

••• (12) •••

Without winter no one would appreciate and love summer so much. Visit the tree that gave you shade during the hot summer and give thanks to its continual seasonal growth.

When the breath wanders, the mind is unsteady, but when the breath is still, so is the mind still.

HATHA YOGA PRADIPIKA

Change procrastination into positive action and feel your emotional energy lighten as a result. Now is the moment of power.

••• 15 •••

Wear leg or arm warmers during your practice to provide additional warmth and to keep the cold away from your wrists and ankles.

Cloves attack germs and are a natural painkiller. Put a clove under your tongue to help rid a sore throat or soothe a toothache.

Twist in Chair to help release stiffness in your back. Start in Chair (see page 95). Inhale and bring hands to Prayer (see page 20). Exhale and bring your right elbow to your left knee. Look skyward. Hold. Breathe. Repeat on the other side.

Exercise your jaw to release stress built up from clenching and gritting your teeth. Close your eyes. Inhale and slowly open your mouth as wide as you can. Exhale and gently close your mouth. Repeat eight times.

There is really no such thing as bad weather, only different kinds of good weather.

JOHN RUSKIN

Increase circulation to your kidneys in Side Open Angle. Sit with your left leg spread as wide as possible, hips facing forward, and your right leg bent inward. Inhale. Exhale and extend your arms, aiming to hold your right foot. Repeat on the other side.

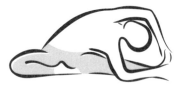

Whenever a pose calls for you to balance on one foot, try this before you lift your leg to help you feel grounded and secure. Start by lifting your toes, spreading them wide apart and then lowering them back onto the mat, becoming aware of each toe on the floor. Then notice the balls of your feet and the soles of your feet as you spread your weight evenly over each foot. Engage your thighs and core, lift your kneecaps and draw the crown of your head to the sky, then lift.

• • • (22) • • •

Put some fresh lavender under your pillow and have an early night. A good night's sleep helps the body to function at its best.

• • • (23) • • •

Collect some delicious, heart-warming soup recipes to comfort and fuel you through the winter.

••• (24) •••

A Shoulder Stand is an ideal pick-me-up. Start in Plough (see page 132). Inhale and slowly bring your legs directly above your head. Support the small of your back with your hands, fingertips pointing skyward. Place a towel underneath you if it helps. Hold. Breathe.

25

Desire, ask, believe, receive.

STELLA TERRILL MANN

••• (26) •••

The normal spine is a gently curved "S" shape naturally designed to distribute the weight of your bones and keep your body upright. Think, "I am long, lovely and erect" whenever you remember today to avoid slumping and slouching into your spine.

••• (27) •••

Take a seated meditation using *Abhaya Mudra*, the hand gesture of fearlessness. Raise your right hand to chest level with your palm facing forward. Extend your fingers skyward with the intention of bringing emotional energy and courage into your heart.

••• (28) •••

To further open the upper chest in Side Angle (see page 86), add a Bind. Take the outstretched arm and reach behind your back to touch the top of the opposite thigh. Hold for as long as is comfortable.

••• •••

Frequently wriggle, waggle, shake and bend your fingers during the day to keep the blood flowing and maintain warmth. They get cold with poor circulation.

••• •••

Head to Knee opens your hips and the backs of your legs, allowing tension to release. Start in Staff (see page 28), then bend your right knee and bring the sole to your thigh. Inhale and lift your arms over your head, lining up your torso with your left leg, then exhale and fold forward. Keep your spine long and chest open, and take hold of the left foot if you can, or your shin if not. Draw your shoulders back and down and breathe into the pose. Repeat on the other side.

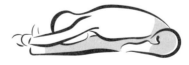

december

After any inversion, when your head has been below your heart (as in Standing Forward Bend, Child and Shoulder Stand), close your eyes as you straighten to avoid a light-headed feeling or dizziness.

You cannot do yoga. Yoga is your natural state. What you can do are yoga exercises, which may reveal to you where you are resisting your natural state.

SHARON GANNON

Contemplate the shape and structure of a naked winter tree to see the similarities between you and a tree: its trunk is your body; its roots your feet; its branches your arms and legs; and its twigs your fingers and toes.

Relax at the end of the day in Frontal Corpse. Lie on your front with your big toes touching. Create a cushion with your hands and lay your head to one side. Breathe.

••• 05 •••

Warm up the tiny muscles in your feet to avoid straining them before slipping into your party shoes. Rotate your ankles, flex and extend your feet. Inhale: lift onto your toes. Exhale: lower down to the floor.

Give yourself a full-body stretch at the end of a
hip-opening session in Mermaid. Start in Pigeon (see
page 128), right leg forward, pressing through the
fingertips to reach your crown to the sky.

Bend your left knee and reach
your left arm back so your foot
is pressing against the inside of
your elbow. Lift your right
arm above you and bend at
the elbow to reach back and
clasp the left hand.

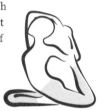

Considered to be the king of *asanas*, a Headstand
requires concentration and enough body strength
to protect the spine. Practise against a wall to
build confidence and seek guidance from your
teacher to avoid injury.

See your extra bags of shopping as a productive workout, rather than a chore. Bone-healing and -strengthening activity is stimulated by carrying and lifting weight.

••• (09) •••

Lie on your back with bent knees to shift a bloated feeling. Inhale. Exhale: bend and wrap your arms around your knees. Slowly squeeze them to your chest. Gently rock forward and backward on your spine to expel any trapped wind.

••• (10) •••

Choose the mantra *ham* (pronounced "h-a-au-m") during meditation to focus your attention on your throat chakra and free your voice. Wear blue, which is the colour associated with the fifth chakra.

Have only love in your heart for others. The more you see the good in them, the more you will establish good in yourself.

PARAMAHANSA YOGANANDA

Visualize yourself surrounded by light to shield your personal energy from the demands of the outside world and the negativity of others.

••• 13 •••

Be the designer of your own life; create dreams and then make them come true. Live your life!

••• (14) •••

We are what our thoughts have made us; so take care about what you think. Words are secondary. Thoughts live; they travel far.

SWAMI VIVEKANANDA

••• (15) •••

Energize your mind in Wheel. Lie on your back. Inhale: bend your knees, placing your feet on the floor as close to your buttocks as possible. Bring your hands under your shoulders, fingers pointing toward your feet. Inhale: lift your body. Hold. Breathe. Lower on an exhalation.

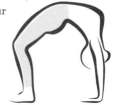

••• (16) •••

Camomile tea is great when drunk hot to soothe a cold. But it can also be used cold: dampen cotton wool pads with cold camomile tea to ease sore eyes if they are inflamed from a lot of sneezing.

••• (17) •••

Keep your levels of vitamin C topped up by eating plenty of fruit to protect you from winter colds and germs.

••• (18) •••

Unwind in a deep hot bath to relax your muscles, reduce cramps and relieve tension headaches. Similar to the effect of a massage, a good hot soak will relax your muscles.

How people treat you is their karma; how you react is yours.

WAYNE DYER

Release energy flow in your spine in Knee to Ear. Start in Plough (see page 132). Inhale. Exhale: bend your knees to your ears. Extend your arms against the floor in the opposite direction to your feet, palms facing down.

••• 21 •••

Lighten up the shortest day of the year with candles and fairy lights. Remind yourself that daylight hours will be a fraction longer tomorrow!

••• 22 •••

Tap into your core strength in Lateral Plank. From Plank (see page 32), inhale and turn on your toes, bringing the outer edge of your right foot to connect with the floor and stacking your left foot on top of it. Lift your left arm skyward. Hold. Breathe. Repeat on the other side.

••• 23 •••

The body makes between one to two litres of saliva daily. Chewing helps to stimulate saliva production within the mouth. Chew your food thoroughly to help the manufacture of this essential digestive juice.

Set an affirmation for the day, week, month or year ahead to make you conscious of positive thought. Create a short powerful statement and assert that what you want to be true is true.

••• 25 •••

Be still in Hero to relieve high blood pressure. Kneel with your feet hip distance apart. Inhale: cross both arms above your head. Exhale: lower your buttocks to the floor. Rest your palms on your knees.

••• 26 •••

Treat yourself to new comfortable yoga clothing or a new yoga mat for the year ahead.

••• (27) •••

Training of mind and body leads to awareness of the soul.

B. K. S. IYENGAR

••• (28) •••

Marichyasana is a great pose for lengthening your hamstrings, opening your hips and stimulating both your abdominal and pelvic region. Start in Staff (see page 28), then bend your right knee and place the foot flat on the mat as close to your buttocks as possible. Exhale as you fold forward, bending your right forearm back to wrap around the outside of your right leg. Reach back with your left arm and take hold of your right wrist. Hold for a few breaths and repeat on the other side.

Look back through your diary to see the changes you have experienced and the positive steps you have made throughout the year. However small or large your steps have been, they all help to create a better you!

••• (30) •••

Take strength from endings as they create space for new beginnings.

••• (31) •••

Namaste – the divine light in me recognizes the divine light in you.

conclusion

You've reached the end of what has hopefully been a fulfilling and prosperous year. This book's aim was for you to make small gains in your yoga journey and to improve your mental and physical health. If you did make more progress in your flexibility, strength and stamina than you thought you would, then that's an added bonus. Although you've come to the end of the book, we hope that you continue practising yoga into the future and refer back to the many wonderful poses and breathing techniques you have learned.

Good luck, enjoy and *namaste*.

notes

....
....
....
....
....
....
....
....
....
....
....
....
....

If you're interested in finding out more
about our books, find us on Facebook
at Summersdale Publishers, on Twitter
at @Summersdale and on Instagram
at @summersdalebooks.

www.summersdale.com